36 Meal Recipes to Help You Prevent Cavities, Gum Disease, Tooth Loss, and Oral Cancer:

The All-Natural Solution to Your Oral Problems

By

Joe Correa CSN

COPYRIGHT

This publication is designed to provide accurate and authoritative information in regard to the subject matter covered. It is sold with the understanding that neither the author nor the publisher is engaged in rendering medical advice. If medical advice or assistance is needed, consult with a doctor. This book is considered a guide and should not be used in any way detrimental to your health. Consult with a physician before starting this nutritional plan to make sure it's right for you.

ACKNOWLEDGEMENTS

This book is dedicated to my friends and family that have had mild or serious illnesses so that you may find a solution and make the necessary changes in your life.

36 Meal Recipes to Help You Prevent Cavities, Gum Disease, Tooth Loss, and Oral Cancer:

The All-Natural Solution to Your Oral Problems

By

Joe Correa CSN

CONTENTS

ABOUT THE AUTHOR

After years of Research, I honestly believe in the positive effects that proper nutrition can have over the body and mind. My knowledge and experience has helped me live healthier throughout the years and which I have shared with family and friends. The more you know about eating and drinking healthier, the sooner you will want to change your life and eating habits.

Nutrition is a key part in the process of being healthy and living longer so get started today. The first step is the most important and the most significant.

INTRODUCTION

36 Meal Recipes to Help You Prevent Cavities, Gum Disease, Tooth Loss, and Oral Cancer: The All-Natural Solution to Your Oral Problems

By Joe Correa CSN

The first thing that comes to mind when you think about oral health is definitely oral hygiene. Without a doubt, this is the main factor responsible for healthy teeth and the best help you can possibly get in preventing any complications. Brushing daily and flossing keeps your teeth and gums healthy and reduces the chances of having cavities. However, even when we follow our dentist's advice, some complications still happen. The number one culprit for this is usually a bad diet.

Having tooth cavities is common all over the world. This bacterial infection destroys teeth and can cause serious pain. Millions of people suffer from this problem and, unfortunately, some of them completely avoid treating it and end up a tooth removed or even worse.

As we already know, the #1 enemy is sugar. This well-known fact is incorporated in many health campaigns and dentist advice but avoiding sugar won't solve your problem completely. Avoiding sugar is just the first step in taking care of your teeth. Other important factors that can negatively affect your oral health are: alcohol, cigarettes, and a poor diet.

Alcohol has a triple impact on your teeth. It's full of sugar that remains in your mouth for a long period of time and it feeds the bad bacteria directly in your mouth. Alcohol also causes dehydration which reduces the healthy flow of saliva. This causes bacteria to stay in your mouth instead of being washed away naturally. Alcohol (just like cigarettes) will leave some nasty stains on your teeth and ruin the nice white color of your teeth.

A lot has been said about the negative effects that cigarettes can have on your teeth. Tobacco limits your mouth's ability to fight off bacteria and infections and it exposes your mouth to tooth decay. Just like alcohol, it leaves those terrible yellow stains on your teeth which are almost impossible to get rid of. Besides, cigarettes are proven to cause many different types of cancer, among those oral cancer.

Nutrition is the single most important factor affecting your oral health after oral hygiene. The answer lies in having a specific diet full of vitamins, minerals, omega-3 fatty acids, and antioxidants that are proven to build up and strengthen your teeth and that's what this book is all about.

These recipes are low in sugar, but extremely rich in other nutrients that will help you to have the smile you've always wanted. Combine them with proper oral hygiene and you'll drastically reduce your chances of having tooth cavities, gum disease, tooth loss, and oral cancer.

36 MEAL RECIPES TO HELP YOU PREVENT CAVITIES, GUM DISEASE, TOOTH LOSS, AND ORAL CANCER: THE ALL-NATURAL SOLUTION TO YOUR ORAL PROBLEMS

1.   Warm Basmati Salad

Ingredients:

2 cups of basmati rice

½ cup of spring onions, chopped

¼ cup of fresh cilantro, finely chopped

4 tbsp of apple cider vinegar

2 tbsp of lemon juice, freshly squeezed

¼ tsp of chili pepper, ground

½ tsp of salt

¼ tsp of black pepper, ground

Preparation:

Place the rice in a deep pot. Add about 4 cups of water and bring it to a boil over medium-high temperature.

Now, reduce the heat and cover with a lid. Cook for about 40-45 minutes, or until soften.

Meanwhile, combine all other ingredients in a large bowl. Add cooked rice and stir all well to combine. Serve immediately.

Nutrition information per serving: Kcal: 463, Protein: 9.2g, Carbs: 100.4g, Fats: 0.9g

2.   Tomato Beef Stew

Ingredients:

2 lbs of lean beef, cut into bite-sized pieces

2 cups of tomatoes, diced

½ cup of celery, chopped

1 cup of potatoes, peeled and chopped

½ cup of red wine vinegar

2 garlic cloves, finely chopped

1 medium-sized onion

2 tbsp of fresh parsley, finely chopped

3 tbsp of olive oil

½ tsp of salt

¼ tsp of black pepper, ground

Preparation:

Preheat the oil in a large skillet over a medium-high temperature. Add meat and 2-3 tablespoons of water to prevent sticking to the skillet. Cook until slightly browned, and then add onions and garlic. Cook for another minute, then add tomatoes, celery, vinegar, parsley, salt, and pepper. Add water to adjust the thickness. Bring it to a boil then reduce the heat to low. Cook for 40 minutes, then add potatoes. Cook for another 20 minutes. Remove from the heat and serve warm.

Nutrition information per serving: Kcal: 230, Protein: 28.3g, Carbs: 5.3g, Fats: 10.0g

3.   Almond Carrot Smoothie

Ingredients:

1 cup of Greek yogurt

2 medium-sized carrots, sliced

1 medium-sized banana, sliced

2 tbsp of almonds, roughly chopped

Preparation:

Combine carrots, banana, and almonds in a food processor. Blend until for 1 minute, then add yogurt and blend for another minute, or until creamy and smooth. Transfer the mixture to a serving glasses and garnish with some extra almonds. Serve immediately.

Nutrition information per serving: Kcal: 180, Protein: 11.5g, Carbs: 24.4g, Fats: 5.0g

4.   Shrimp Pasta

Ingredients:

1 lb of pasta, whole wheat

2 lbs of shrimps, cleaned and deveined

1 lb of bell peppers, seeded and chopped

3 garlic cloves, crushed

4 tbsp of olive oil

1 large lemon, juiced

1 tsp of lemon zest

½ tsp of sea salt

¼ tsp of black pepper, freshly ground

Preparation:

Preheat the oil in a large nonstick pan over a medium-high temperature. Add garlic and stir-fry for 5 minutes, or until translucent. Now, add shrimps and peppers. Cook for 3-4 minutes then add lemon juice. Sprinkle with some salt and pepper. Cook for a few minutes more, or until heated trough. Remove from the heat and set aside.

Cook pasta using package instructions. Drain well and transfer to a large bowl. Add shrimps and toss to combine. Serve immediately.

Nutrition information per serving: Kcal: 367, Protein: 32.6g, Carbs: 35.0g, Fats: 10.3g

5. Honey-Herb Turkey

Ingredients:

2 lbs of turkey breasts, thinly sliced

2 garlic cloves, minced

4 tbsp of orange juice

1 tsp of fresh sage, finely chopped

1 tsp of dried thyme, ground

2 tbsp of olive oil

½ cup of honey, raw

¼ tsp of salt

¼ tsp of black pepper, ground

Preparation:

Combine orange juice, sage, thyme, garlic, salt, and pepper in a medium bowl. Stir well and set aside.

Grease a large baking dish with olive oil. Spread the turkey breasts in a dish and pour the half of the honey mixture. Place it in the oven and bake for 30 minutes. Turn over the breasts and add the remaining mixture. Bake for about 25 minutes more. Remove from the heat and serve.

Nutrition information per serving: Kcal: 290, Protein: 26.1g, Carbs: 31.3g, Fats: 7.2g

6.   Cheese Tomato Omelet

Ingredients:

6 large eggs

½ cup of goat's cheese, crumbled

½ cup of cherry tomatoes, diced

1 tbsp of skim milk

3 garlic cloves, minced

1 tbsp of olive oil

½ tsp of salt

¼ tsp of black pepper, ground

Preparation:

Combine eggs, cheese, milk, salt, and pepper in a mixing bowl. Whisk well and set aside.

Preheat the oil in a large frying pan over a medium-high temperature. Add garlic and stir-fry for about 3-4 minutes, or until translucent. Add tomatoes and cook for 2 minutes. Pour the egg mixture and stir once. Cook for 2 minutes, then flip the omelet. Cook for another 2 minutes and remove from the heat. Fold the omelet in half and serve.

Nutrition information per serving: Kcal: 438, Protein: 28.5g, Carbs: 6.0g, Fats: 34.0g

7.   Artichoke Pesto Pasta

Ingredients:

1 cup of artichokes, chopped

1 lb of pasta, pre-cooked

½ cup of Parmesan cheese, grated

2 tbsp of Pecan nuts, roughly chopped

2 garlic cloves, minced

1 cup of fresh basil, chopped

½ cup of parsley, chopped

1 lemon, juiced

4 tbsp of olive oil

½ tsp of kosher salt

¼ tsp of black pepper, ground

Preparation:

Place artichokes in a pot of boiling water. Cook until slightly soften and remove from the heat. Drain well and set aside.

Cook the pasta using package instructions. Drain and transfer to a serving plate.

Meanwhile, combine cheese, nuts, basil, parsley, oil, lemon juice, salt, pepper, and garlic in a food processor. Blend until nice and creamy. Now, add artichokes and re-blend for 1 minute until all well incorporated. Stir in the desired amount of mixture into the pasta and store the rest in a jar and refrigerate.

Nutrition information per serving: Kcal: 586, Protein: 21.8g, Carbs: 69.7g, Fats: 26.1g

8.   Spinach Shitake Mushrooms

Ingredients:

2 cups of fresh spinach, chopped

1 cup of Shitake mushrooms, chopped

1 cup of button mushrooms, chopped

½ cup of cherry tomatoes, chopped

1 cup of Iceberg lettuce, chopped

½ cup of green olives, pitted and halved

2 garlic cloves, minced

4 tbsp of lime juice, freshly squeezed

1 tsp of lime zest

2 tbsp of butter

3 tbsp of extra-virgin olive oil

½ tsp of sea salt

¼ tsp of black pepper, ground

Preparation:

Now, mix together lime juice, vinegar, mustard, oil, salt, and pepper in a mixing bowl. Set aside to allow flavors to mingle.

Melt 1 tablespoon of butter in a medium nonstick saucepan over a medium-high temperature. Add Shitake, button mushrooms and 2 tablespoons of water to prevent sticking to the pan. Cook for 7-10 minutes, or until tender. Transfer the mushrooms to a large salad bowl and reserve the pan.

Melt the remaining butter and add garlic. Stir-fry until translucent. throw in the spinach and cook for 3-4 minutes, or until tender. Remove from the heat and transfer to the bowl with mushrooms.

Now, add tomatoes, lettuce, and olives. Stir once, then drizzle all with previously made dressing. Toss to coat well. Serve immediately.

Nutrition information per serving: Kcal: 252, Protein: 2.8g, Carbs: 12.9g, Fats: 23.2g

9.   Avocado Kale Salad

Ingredients:

1 medium-sized avocado, pitted, peeled and chopped

2 cups of fresh kale, chopped

2 tbsp of lemon juice, freshly squeezed

4 tbsp of orange juice, freshly squeezed

2 tbsp of almonds, roughly chopped

2 tbsp of olive oil

¼ tsp of salt

¼ tsp of black pepper, ground

Preparation:

Combine lemon juice, orange juice, almonds, oil, salt, and pepper in a mixing bowl. Mix well and set aside.

Place kale in a deep pot of boiling water. Sprinkle with some salt and cook for 10 minutes, or until crisp. If you like it more tender, then cook for 20 minutes.

Remove from the heat and drain well. Set aside to cool completely.

Now, combine chopped avocado and kale in a medium salad bowl. Drizzle with the dressing and toss to coat. Garnish with lemon wedges and serve.

Nutrition information per serving: Kcal: 411, Protein: 5.5g, Carbs: 20.6g, Fats: 36.8g

10.   Chicken Basil Pesto

Ingredients:

1 lb of chicken fillets, chopped

1 cup of fresh basil, chopped

4 tbsp of olive oil

¼ cup of tomatoes, sun-dried

2 garlic cloves, minced

3 tbsp of lemon juice, freshly squeezed

¼ tsp of sea salt

¼ tsp of black pepper, ground

Preparation:

Combine all ingredients except olive oil in a food processor and blend for 1 minute, or until nicely incorporated. Gradually add 2 tablespoons of oil and blend again. Set aside.

Preheat the remaining oil in a large nonstick frying pan over a medium-high temperature. add chicken and sprinkle with some salt. Cook for 5 minutes, or until golden brown. Transfer the chicken to a serving plate and spoon the pesto on top. Serve immediately.

Nutrition information per serving: Kcal: 459, Protein: 44.4g, Carbs: 1.9g, Fats: 30.1g

11.   Beef with Milk Peppers

Ingredients:

1 lbs of beef, cut into bite-sized pieces

½ cup of vegetable broth

2 large bell peppers, chopped

2 tbsp of skim milk

3 garlic cloves, minced

1 large red onion, chopped

2 tbsp of olive oil

1 tsp of Himalayan salt

¼ tsp of black pepper, ground

Preparation:

Preheat the oil in a large nonstick saucepan over a medium high temperature.

Add the meat and cook for 5 minutes, then add vegetable broth. Cook until the liquid evaporates, or until the meat softens. Transfer the meat to a serving plate and reserve the pan.

Add garlic and onion and stir-fry for 3 minutes, or until translucent. Add peppers and sprinkle with salt and pepper to taste. Cook for 3 minutes then add milk. Cook until milk heated trough and remove from the heat. Serve peppers with meat.

Nutrition information per serving: Kcal: 253, Protein: 29.1g, Carbs: 7.5g, Fats: 11.6g

12.   Creamy Egg Soup

Ingredients:

3 large eggs

4 cups of chicken broth

1 small carrot, sliced

1 cup of cream cheese

2 tbsp of fresh parsley, finely chopped

1 cup of spring onions, chopped

1 tbsp of cornstarch

¼ tsp of salt

¼ tsp of Cayenne pepper, ground

¼ tsp of salt

Preparation:

Whisk eggs, salt, and pepper in a small bowl and set aside.

Pour the broth into a heavy-bottomed pot. Bring it to a boil and then add cornstarch, carrot, and spring onions. Reduce the heat to low and cover with a lid. Cook for 2 more minutes. Remove from the heat and stir in the cream cheese, parsley, and Cayenne pepper.

Serve warm and reheat the soup if needed.

Nutrition information per serving: Kcal: 181, Protein: 8.3g, Carbs: 4.5g, Fats: 14.5g

13. Broccoli and Cheddar Cheese

Ingredients:

4 cups of broccoli, chopped

1 cup of cheddar cheese, crumbled

1 small onion, finely chopped

4 large eggs

1 cup of skim milk

1 tbsp of olive oil

½ tsp of salt

¼ tsp of black pepper, ground

Preparation:

Preheat the oven to 375°F.

Take a medium baking dish and place some baking paper. Grease with 1 tablespoon of oil and set aside.

Preheat the remaining oil in a large nonstick frying pan over a medium-high temperature. Add broccoli and about 2-3 tablespoons of water to prevent sticking to the pan. Cook for about 7-8 minutes, or until tender. When done, remove from the pan and drain well. Set aside.

Meanwhile, combine eggs, milk, and cheese. Stir well to blend and transfer it to a bowl with broccoli. Give it a good stir and pour the mixture into the baking dish.

Now, take a large baking dish, and pour water in it (about 1 inch will be enough). Place the baking dish in it and place all in the oven. Bake for about 45-50 minutes, or until the toothpick comes out clean after inserted.

Remove from the oven and let it cool for a while. Serve warm.

Nutrition information per serving: Kcal: 221, Protein: 14.5g, Carbs: 9.2g, Fats: 14.5g

14. Kiwi Strawberry Smoothie

Ingredients:

3 large kiwis, peeled and chopped

¼ cup of strawberries, chopped

1 medium-sized banana, chopped

1 cup of Greek yogurt

1 tbsp of honey, raw

Preparation:

Combine all ingredients in a food processor and blend until nicely smooth and creamy. Transfer to a serving glasses and garnish with some nuts or seeds. However, this is optional. Refrigerate for 20 minutes before serving.

Nutrition information per serving: Kcal: 172, Protein: 8.2g, Carbs: 23.0g, Fats: 1.9g

15.   Wild Salmon & Veggie Puree

Ingredients:

2 lbs of wild salmon filets, boneless, thinly sliced

2 cups of sweet potatoes, peeled and chopped

1 small red bell pepper, finely chopped

1 small green pepper, finely chopped

1 tbsp of fresh parsley, finely chopped

4 tbsp of olive oil

2 garlic cloves

1 small red onion, finely chopped

1 tsp of fresh rosemary, finely chopped

1 tsp of sea salt

½ tsp of black pepper, freshly ground

Preparation:

Place potatoes in a pot of boiling water and cook until fork-tender. Remove from the heat and drain well.

Transfer to a food processor and sprinkle with salt. Blend until smooth and place it in a bowl. Add chopped red bell pepper, green bell pepper, red onion, and parsley. Stir all to combine and set aside.

Preheat 2 tablespoons of oil in a large frying pan over a medium-high temperature. Add garlic and stir-fry for 2 minutes and then add meat. Cook for 3 minutes on each side, or until golden crisp. Remove from the heat and set aside.

Mix together the remaining oil, rosemary, salt, and pepper in a small bowl.

Place salmon and potato puree on a serving plate. Drizzle with marinade and serve immediately.

Nutrition information per serving: Kcal: 355, Protein: 30.6g, Carbs: 17.7g, Fats: 18.9g

16.   Ginger Apple Oatmeal

Ingredients:

1 cup of green apples, cut into bite-sized pieces

1 cup of oatmeal

1 cup of skim milk

½ tsp of ginger, ground

1 tbsp of honey, raw

1 tbsp of flaxseeds

Preparation:

Place apples in a pot of boiling water and cook until soft tender. Remove from the heat and drain well. Combine cooked apples, oatmeal, and milk in a deep pot. Cook for 3 minutes, or until heated through. Remove from the heat and stir in the honey. Spoon into serving bowls and top with flaxseeds before serving.

Nutrition information per serving: Kcal: 310, Protein: 10.4g, Carbs: 59.1g, Fats: 4.0g

17. Turkey Casserole

Ingredients:

1 lb of turkey breasts, skinless and boneless

½ cup of Parmesan cheese, grated

½ cup of chicken broth

1 small carrot, chopped

1 medium-sized tomato, diced

1 tbsp of sour cream

2 tbsp of olive oil

1 tbsp of fresh parsley, finely chopped

1 tbsp of fresh celery, finely chopped

1 tsp of dried thyme, ground

¼ tsp of red pepper flakes

½ tsp of salt

Preparation:

Preheat the oven to 375°F.

Place some baking paper in a casserole dish and sprinkle with some cooking spray.

Preheat the oil in a frying pan over a medium-high temperature. add carrots and cook for 3 minutes, or until slightly tender. Now, add meat and stir in the tomato. Sprinkle with some salt and cook for 5 minutes, then remove from the heat and transfer to a prepared casserole dish. Season with parsley, celery, thyme, salt, and red pepper. Pour the vegetable broth and spread the cheese. Place it in the oven and bake for 20-25 minutes. Remove from the oven and cut into portions. Top with sour cream and serve.

Nutrition information per serving: Kcal: 266, Protein: 26.9g, Carbs: 8.5g, Fats: 14.1g

18.   Pasta Marinara

Ingredients:

2 lbs of pasta

1 large bell pepper, chopped

1 cup of tomatoes, diced

½ cup of tomato paste

1 small onion, finely chopped

2 garlic cloves, minced

1 tbsp of olive oil

1 tbsp of fresh parsley, finely chopped

½ tsp of chili pepper, ground

1 tsp of dried oregano, ground

½ tsp of sea salt

Preparation:

Cook pasta using package instructions. Remove from the heat and drain well. Set aside.

Meanwhile, preheat the oil in a large skillet over a medium-high temperature. Add garlic, onion, and pepper.

Sprinkle with some salt to taste. Cook until browned and stir in the tomatoes, parsley, oregano, and chili. Cook for 2 minutes stirring constantly. Now, add tomato sauce and stir until it boils. Remove from the heat and combine with pasta. Toss to coat well and serve.

Nutrition information per serving: Kcal: 492, Protein: 18.8g, Carbs: 91.2g, Fats: 6.1g

19.   Vegetable Tuna Salad

Ingredients:

1 lbs of tuna, minced

1 cup of Iceberg lettuce, chopped

1 small carrot, sliced

1 small onion, finely chopped

¼ cup of cucumber, cubed

1 small red bell pepper, cubed

2 tbsp of extra-virgin olive oil

1 tbsp of fresh parsley, finely chopped

3 tbsp of lemon juice, freshly squeezed

½ tsp of sea salt

¼ tsp of black pepper, ground

Preparation:

Mix together oil, lemon juice, parsley, salt, and pepper in a small bowl. Stir well and set aside to allow flavors to meld.

Meanwhile, combine tuna, carrot, onion, cucumber, and bell pepper in a large bowl. Stir well and drizzle with previously made marinade. Toss all again to coat. Serve immediately.

Nutrition information per serving: Kcal: 299, Protein: 30.9g, Carbs: 6.1g, Fats: 16.4g

20.   Quick Creamy Omelet

Ingredients:

5 large eggs

3 tbsp of sour cream

1 tbsp of fresh parsley, finely chopped

2 tbsp of chives, chopped

1 tbsp of butter

½ tsp of kosher salt

¼ tsp of black pepper, ground

Preparation:

Combine eggs, parsley, chives, salt, and pepper in a medium bowl. Whisk well with a fork and set aside.

Melt the butter in a nonstick frying pan over a medium-low temperature. Pour the egg mixture and cook for 3-5 minutes, stirring constantly. Remove from the heat and stir in the cream. Serve immediately.

Nutrition information per serving: Kcal: 150, Protein: 16.6g, Carbs: 2.1g, Fats: 22.0g

21.   Almond Coconut Cereals

Ingredients:

½ cup of coconut, shredded

1 cup of flaked almonds

1 large banana, sliced

½ cup of almond milk

½ cup of fresh strawberries, chopped

¼ tsp of cinnamon, ground

1 tsp of coconut oil, melted

1 tbsp of liquid honey

Preparation:

Preheat the oven to 300°F.

Combine coconut, almonds, cinnamon, and melted coconut oil.

Spread some parchment paper in a baking dish. Spread the mixture evenly and place it in the oven. Bake for 3 minutes and remove from the oven. Do not overburn. Set aside to cool for a while.

Meanwhile, combine milk, strawberries, banana, and honey in a bowl. Pour this mixture on top of the coconut mixture. Set aside to cool completely and refrigerate for 30 minutes before serving.

Nutrition information per serving: Kcal: 608, Protein: 13.1g, Carbs: 43.7g, Fats: 47.3g

22.   Green Beans Salad

Ingredients:

3 cups of green beans, pre-cooked

3 oz of Feta cheese, crumbled

½ cup of tomatoes, chopped

¼ cup of shallots, chopped

2 tbsp of olive oil

2 tbsp of balsamic vinegar

3 tbsp of fresh basil, chopped

½ tsp of sea salt

¼ tsp of black pepper, ground

Preparation:

Place the beans in a pot of boiling water. Cook until beans tender, then remove from the heat. Drain well and set aside to cool.

Meanwhile, combine oil, vinegar, basil, salt and pepper. Stir well and set aside.

In a large bowl, combine cheese, tomatoes, shallots, and previously cooked beans. Drizzle with dressing and toss to coat. Serve immediately.

Nutrition information per serving: Kcal: 207, Protein: 6.7g, Carbs: 12.7g, Fats: 15.6g

23. Cranberries Beet Smoothie

Ingredients:

1 cup of fresh cranberries

½ cup of beets, trimmed and pre-cooked

½ cup of spinach, chopped

1 cup of skim milk

1 tsp of fresh mint, chopped

1 tbsp of liquid honey

Preparation:

Place beets in a pot of boiling water and cook until fork-tender. remove from the heat and drain. Set aside to cool completely, or rinse under cold water and drain again.

Now, combine cooked beets, cranberries, spinach, milk, and honey in a food processor. Blend until smooth and transfer to a serving glasses. Garnish with mint and refrigerate for 1 hour before serving.

Nutrition information per serving: Kcal: 128, Protein: 5.0g, Carbs: 24.2g, Fats: 0.1g

24. Veal Steak with Root Vegetables

Ingredients:

2 lbs of veal steaks

½ cup of celery, chopped

2 large carrots, sliced

½ cup of kohlrabi, trimmed and chopped

¼ cup of fresh parsley, finely chopped

2 tbsp of olive oil

1 tsp of balsamic vinegar

1 tbsp of sour cream

¼ tsp of Cayenne pepper, ground

¼ tsp of black pepper, ground

½ tsp of sea salt

2 tbsp of lemon juice, freshly squeezed

1 tsp of fresh rosemary, finely chopped

Preparation:

Preheat the oven to 425°F.

Combine celery, carrots, kohlrabi, in a pot of boiling water and cook for about 5 minutes, or until tender. Transfer the vegetables to a large baking dish. Drizzle with vinegar, Cayenne pepper, salt and brush with 1 tablespoon of oil. Bake for 3-5 minutes, or until crisp. Remove from the heat and set aside to cool.

Preheat the remaining oil in a large frying pan and add veal steaks. Sprinkle with some salt and cook for 8-10 minutes on both sides, or until golden brown. Remove from the heat and set aside.

Transfer the meat and vegetables to a serving plate. Drizzle with lemon juice and sprinkle with rosemary before serving.

Nutrition information per serving: Kcal: 327, Protein: 40.4g, Carbs: 3.9g, Fats: 15.7g

25.   Chicken Zucchini

Ingredients:

1 lb of chicken breasts, skinless and boneless

2 large zucchinis, peeled and chopped

2 garlic cloves, minced

1 small onion, chopped

4 tbsp of olive oil

½ tsp of kosher salt

¼ tsp of black pepper, ground

Preparation:

Place the zucchinis in a pot of boiling water and cook for 2 minutes. Remove from the heat and drain well. Set aside.

Preheat the oil in a large skillet over a medium-high temperature. Add garlic and onion, and stir-fry for about 1 minute. Add meat and cook for 7-10 minutes or until golden brown. Now, add zucchinis and sprinkle with some salt and pepper. Cook for about 2-4 minutes and remove from the heat. Serve chicken with zucchinis.

Nutrition information per serving: Kcal: 247, Protein: 23.4g, Carbs: 5.1g, Fats: 15.1g

26.   Brown Rice with Cheese Sauce

Ingredients:

1 cup of cherry tomatoes, diced

1 cup of brown rice, long-grained

1 cup of Mozzarella cheese, crumbled

1 small onion, chopped

1 tsp of dried oregano, ground

3 tbsp of basil, finely chopped

2 tbsp of balsamic vinegar

2 tbsp of olive oil

½ tsp of salt

¼ tsp of black pepper, ground

Preparation:

Place the rice in a deep pot. Add 2 ½ cups of water and bring it to a boil. Sprinkle with some salt and reduce the heat to low. Cover with a lid and cook for 15 minutes. Remove from the heat and drain the excessive liquid. Set aside to cool completely.

Now, preheat 1 tablespoon of oil in a saucepan over a medium-high temperature. Add onion and stir-fry until translucent. Add tomatoes and cheese and cook until cheese melts. Remove from the heat and stir in the vinegar, oregano, basil, salt, pepper, and remaining oil. Combine rice with this mixture and toss well until incorporated.

Serve immediately.

Nutrition information per serving: Kcal: 361, Protein: 8.4g, Carbs: 53.7g, Fats: 12.9g

27.   Shitake Omelet

Ingredients:

4 large eggs

1 cup of shitake mushrooms, chopped

½ cup of Gouda cheese, roughly grated

1 tbsp of butter

½ tsp of Himalayan pink salt

¼ tsp of black pepper, ground

Preparation:

Whisk the eggs, salt, and pepper in a mixing bowl. Set aside.

Melt the butter in a large frying pan over a medium-high temperature. Add mushrooms and cook for about 8-10 minutes, or until soften. Now, sprinkle with grated cheese and cook for another minute, stirring occasionally. Pour the egg mixture and cook for 3-4 minutes, then flip the omelet. Cook for 2 minutes and remove from the heat. Fold the omelet using a spatula and serve.

Sprinkle with some extra cheese and garnish with fresh parsley.

Nutrition information per serving: Kcal: 412, Protein: 26.3g, Carbs: 12.1g, Fats: 29.6g

28.   Veal Bean Stew

Ingredients:

1 lb of lean veal, cut into bite-sized pieces

1 cup of kidney beans

1 cup of chicken broth

2 small onions, chopped

2 cups of tomatoes, diced

3 tbsp of tomato paste

1 medium-sized bell pepper, diced

2 garlic cloves, crushed

2 tbsp of olive oil

1 tsp of chili pepper, ground

½ tsp of dried thyme, ground

½ tsp of dried oregano, ground

½ tsp of cumin, ground

½ tsp of salt

Preparation:

Preheat the oil in a large nonstick skillet over a medium-high temperature. Add the meat and cook until nicely browned. Now, add onion, garlic and diced bell pepper. Stir and cook for 3 minutes. Add diced tomatoes, and tomato paste. Pour the chicken broth and sprinkle with chili, thyme, oregano, cumin, and salt. Stir all well and cook for about 30-35 minutes. Add water to adjust thickness while cooking. Stir in the beans and cook for 10 more minutes. Remove from the heat and serve warm.

Nutrition information per serving: Kcal: 316, Protein: 27.6g, Carbs: 27.1g, Fats: 11.2g

29.   Grilled Eel

Ingredients:

1 lb of eel, cleaned and cut into bite-sized pieces

4 tbsp of olive oil

2 garlic cloves, crushed

1 small onion, chopped

¼ tsp of Cayenne pepper, ground

4 tbsp of white wine vinegar

1 tbsp of butter

1 tsp of seafood seasoning mix

1 cup of all-purpose flour

1 tsp of fresh rosemary, finely chopped

½ tsp of salt

¼ tsp of black pepper, ground

Preparation:

Combine oil, Cayenne pepper, vinegar, seafood seasoning mix, rosemary, salt, and pepper in a medium bowl. Place the eel chunks in this mixture and toss well to coat. Set aside for 1 hour to allow flavors to penetrate into the meat.

Melt the butter in a large nonstick frying pan over a medium-high temperature. Now, spread the flour on a clean kitchen surface. Spoon the eel on it, draining the marinade. Coat with flour and place it in the frying pan. Fry for 5 minutes, then add onion and garlic. Now, add ½ cup of water and the remaining marinade. Cook for the next 10 minutes, or until the liquid reduced by half.

Remove from the heat and serve immediately.

Nutrition information per serving: Kcal: 541, Protein: 30.4g, Carbs: 26.4g, Fats: 34.2g

30.   Carrot Frittata

Ingredients:

3 large carrots, sliced

6 large eggs

1 cup of spring onions, chopped

2 garlic cloves, minced

½ cup of Gouda cheese, shredded

½ cup of fresh celery, chopped

1 tbsp of olive oil

2 tsp of butter

¼ tsp of dried oregano, ground

½ tsp of kosher salt

¼ tsp of black pepper, ground

Preparation:

Preheat the broiler over a medium-high temperature.

Place the carrots in a pot of boiling water. Add a pinch of salt and cook until tender. Remove from the heat and drain well. Set aside.

Preheat the oil in a large nonstick skillet over a medium-high temperature. Add carrots, spring onions, and garlic. Sprinkle with some salt and pepper and cook for 5 minutes. Remove from the heat and transfer the vegetables to a bowl, but reserve the pan.

Melt the butter in the same skillet over a medium-high temperature.

Meanwhile, mix together eggs, oregano and celery. Season with a pinch of salt and whisk well with a fork. Pour the mixture into the skillet and cook for 3-4 minutes, or until eggs are set. Remove from the heat and top with carrot mixture. Spread the grated cheese and place it under the broiler. Broil for 1 minutes on high until golden brown. Remove and set aside to cool for a while. Serve.

Nutrition information per serving: Kcal: 260, Protein: 15.6g, Carbs: 9.2g, Fats: 18.5g

31.   Raspberry Porridge

Ingredients:

1 cup of rolled oats

1 cup of almond milk

1 cup of water

¼ cup of fresh raspberries

1 large banana, chopped

1 tbsp of sunflower seeds

Preparation:

Pour the water in a medium pot and bring it to a boil. Add oats and cook for 3 minutes, stirring constantly. Remove from the heat and let it soak for 10 minutes.

Now, stir in the almond milk and cook for 1 minute, or until heated trough. Remove from the heat and stir in chopped banana. Top with raspberries and sunflower seeds before serving.

Nutrition information per serving: Kcal: 339, Protein: 6.2g, Carbs: 34.6g, Fats: 21.6g

32.   Beef Burgers

Ingredients:

1 lb of ground beef

1 small onion

¼ tsp of chili pepper, ground

1 tbsp of tomato paste

1 tbsp of fresh parsley, finely chopped

1 tbsp of all-purpose flour

1 garlic clove, minced

¼ tsp of dried oregano, ground

¼ tsp of salt

1 tbsp of sour cream

4 hamburger buns, whole grain

1 tsp of butter

Preparation:

Combine meat, chili, onion, tomato paste, garlic, flour, oregano, salt, and pepper in a large bowl. Mix all with hands and shape the burgers.

Melt the butter in a nonstick skillet over a medium-high temperature. Cook for 6-7 minutes, or until nicely browned. Remove from the heat and set aside.

Place the buns in a toaster and toast for 1 minute. Place the burger on a bottom bun and top with sour cream. Sprinkle with some parsley and cover with a top bun.

Nutrition information per serving: Kcal: 365, Protein: 39.2g, Carbs: 25.7g, Fats: 10.6g

33. Apple Chia Smoothie

Ingredients:

1 large green apple, cored and chopped

1 cup of skim milk

1 large banana, sliced

¼ tsp of cinnamon

1 tbsp of honey, raw

1 tbsp of chia seeds

Preparation:

Combine all ingredients in a food processor. Blend until creamy and smooth. Transfer to a serving glasses and refrigerate for 30 minutes before serving. Enjoy!

Nutrition information per serving: Kcal: 196, Protein: 5.1g, Carbs: 45.8g, Fats: 0.4g

34.   Cremini Mushroom Polenta

Ingredients:

2 cups of cornstarch

¼ cup of shallots, chopped

2 garlic cloves, crushed

1 lb of cremini mushrooms, thinly sliced

1 tsp of salt

¼ tsp of black pepper, ground

Preparation:

Pour 6 cups of water in a heavy-bottomed pot. Bring it to a boil and gently stir in the cornstarch. Cook for 25 minutes, or until mixture thickens, stirring constantly. Remove from the heat and set aside.

Throw in the onion and shallots in a large nonstick skillet over a medium-high temperature. Cook for 1 minute and then add mushrooms and 3-4 tablespoons of water to prevent sticking to the pan. Sprinkle with salt and pepper and cook for 10 minutes, or until tender.

Serve previously cooked polenta and top with mushrooms. Sprinkle with parsley or top with heavy cream. However, this is optional.

Nutrition information per serving: Kcal: 196, Protein: 5.1g, Carbs: 45.8g, Fats: 0.4g

35.   Stuffed Tomatoes

Ingredients:

4 large tomatoes

¼ cup of leeks, diced

1 cup of brown rice

1 small zucchini, peeled and chopped

3 tbsp of fresh basil, chopped

¼ cup of frozen corn, thawed

2 garlic cloves, minced

4 tbsp of lemon juice, freshly squeezed

½ tsp of salt

¼ tsp of black pepper, ground

Preparation:

Preheat the oven to 350°F.

Place the rice in a deep pot and add 3 cups of water. Bring it to a boil and cook for 15 minutes, or until tender. Remove from the heat and set aside.

Combine leeks, garlic, and 2 tablespoons of water in a large nonstick skillet over a medium-high temperature. Cook for 10 minutes, or until tender. Add zucchini and corn. Stir well and cook for another 2-3 minutes.

Stir in the rice, lemon juice, and basil. Sprinkle with some salt and pepper and cook for 1 minute. Remove from the heat and set aside to cool.

Meanwhile, prepare tomatoes. Cut the top and scoop the flesh. Spoon the mixture to prepared tomatoes. Spread the stuffed tomatoes in a large greased baking dish and bake for about 25-30 minutes.

Nutrition information per serving: Kcal: 228, Protein: 6.2g, Carbs: 47.8g, Fats: 2.0g

36.   Vegetarian Eggplant Steaks

Ingredients:

1 large eggplant, thinly sliced

4 tbsp of lemon juice, freshly squeezed

3 tbsp of balsamic vinegar

3 tbsp of heavy cream

1 cup of arugula, roughly chopped

¼ tsp of black pepper, ground

½ tsp of sea salt

¼ tsp of lemon zest

Preparation:

Preheat the grill to a medium-high temperature.

In a mixing bowl, combine lemon juice, heavy cream, vinegar, and sprinkle with some salt and pepper. Dip the eggplant slices in this marinade and place it on the grill.

Grill for 5 minutes on each side, or until doneness.

Spread the sheet of arugula on a serving plate. Top with grilled eggplants and sprinkle with lemon zest before serving.

Nutrition information per serving: Kcal: 100, Protein: 2.2g, Carbs: 10.3g, Fats: 6.0g

ADDITIONAL TITLES FROM THIS AUTHOR

70 Effective Meal Recipes to Prevent and Solve Being Overweight: Burn Fat Fast by Using Proper Dieting and Smart Nutrition

By

Joe Correa CSN

48 Acne Solving Meal Recipes: The Fast and Natural Path to Fixing Your Acne Problems in Less Than 10 Days!

By

Joe Correa CSN

41 Alzheimer's Preventing Meal Recipes: Reduce or Eliminate Your Alzheimer's Condition in 30 Days or Less!

By

Joe Correa CSN

70 Effective Breast Cancer Meal Recipes: Prevent and Fight Breast Cancer with Smart Nutrition and Powerful Foods

By

Joe Correa CSN

www.ingramcontent.com/pod-product-compliance
Lightning Source LLC
Chambersburg PA
CBHW051038030426
42336CB00015B/2931